Mirtha María Peláez Vega

ISCHEMIC STROKE REHABILITATION

Mirtha María Peláez Vega

ISCHEMIC STROKE REHABILITATION

An educational intervention approach for older adults

ScienciaScripts

Imprint

Cover image: www.ingimage.com

This book is a translation from the original published under ISBN 978-613-9-06149-5.

Publisher:
Sciencia Scripts
is a trademark of
Dodo Books Indian Ocean Ltd. and OmniScriptum S.R.L publishing group

120 High Road, East Finchley, London, N2 9ED, United Kingdom
Str. Armeneasca 28/1, office 1, Chisinau MD-2012, Republic of Moldova, Europe
Printed at: see last page
ISBN: 978-620-7-87298-5

Ischemic Stroke Rehabilitation

An Educational Intervention Approach for Older Adults

MIRTHA MARÍA PELÁEZ VEGA

2024

INDEX

INTRODUCTION

For a long time there were people who realized the need for humanity to consider a new form of knowledge of the world and so began to appear the first written testimonies of physical medicine in Greece, Rome, China, and other western European territories that were the background that led to the emergence of this science.

In feudal and capitalist societies, since their origin, they did not pay much attention to the training of scientists that would make possible the scientific education of the time, that is why physiatry was developed by few scientists, which gave rise to the first modalities of rehabilitation, had its emergence empirically, gradually demonstrating in practice its undisputed effectiveness in the motor and psychological reeducation of patients with neurological disorders and the theoretical bases of their techniques were appearing later.

In the 1940s, neurophysiologist Dr. Herman Kabat devised a method of proprioceptive neuromuscular facilitation (PNF), aimed at the neuromuscular system for patients with neurological disorders, using superficial (tactile) and deep proprioceptive information (joint position, tendon and muscle stretching) to excite the nervous system in order to increase muscle strength and coordination. It is mainly used in isotonic or isometric contractions; to strengthen weak muscles; and to stabilize the tone, as well as to give speed to the movement in cases prone to slowness. This method maintains its validity with its closest followers and collaborators, Drs. Knott and Voss (1974) published the book "Proprioceptive Neuromuscular Facilitation, about the original method".

It is considered that these activities must have the active participation of the patient in order to automate the new motor patterns. The most widespread method used in Europe in the last 60 years was developed by Dr. Bobath in 1940, for the treatment of cerebral palsy (CP) and hemiplegia in adults; he considered that the concept of neuro-evolutionary treatment, assumes that the injury during brain maturation, causes a delay or interruption of motor development and abnormal patterns in posture and movements. It is essentially aimed at inhibition of abnormal movement patterns and simultaneous facilitation of the reflex activities of normal patterns.

This method was radically opposed by Dr. Brunnstrom's movement therapy theory, developed specifically for patients with cerebrovascular disease, which postulates that reflexes and synergisms that occur after injury constitute normal recovery patterns and should be stimulated.

The rehabilitation boom in Latin America began after the two world wars, especially the second one and also motivated by the poliomyelitis epidemics of the 40's and 50's. It was logical then, that the first physicians concerned with rehabilitation were orthopedists, due to the need to treat musculoskeletal sequelae that almost always ended in deformities that were surgically resolved. It was logical then, that the first physicians concerned with rehabilitation were orthopedists, due to the need to treat musculoskeletal sequelae that almost always ended in deformities of surgical resolution. They were the initiators of rehabilitation in almost all countries.

One of the main problems of international health systems is to ensure that the rehabilitation of hemiplegic patients who have suffered a cerebrovascular accident (CVA) is really effective. Neurological alterations are usually disabling, caused by different alterations that are part of a cascade of events, triggered by the manifestations of CNS dysfunction.

To develop a specialized rehabilitation, so that patients can develop in their social environment with a better quality of life; that they are able to put into practice their knowledge and skills to face and provide solutions to the problems they face, in coexistence with their disease, and the support of their family, being the patient the protagonist of their rehabilitation process.

Rehabilitation is a therapeutic option to be considered, applicable at any stage of this disease, potentially combinable with any of the other therapeutic variants, offering an additive effect, since its mechanism of action is different from that of drugs or surgery.

Several researchers have contributed conceptualizations on rehabilitation González and Kindelán Alonso (1997) define in their book "Medical Rehabilitation" that it is the restoration of the invalid to his or her maximum possible physical, mental, social, vocational and economic limits.

The World Health Organization (WHO) defines rehabilitation as a process of limited duration, with a defined objective, aimed at enabling persons with impairments or disabilities to attain a functionally optimal physical, mental or social level by providing them with the means to modify their own lives (WHO, 1979).

There is a tendency to consider the rehabilitation of these patients as a process that implies a high consumption of resources, time and effort, requiring for its development a technology that can only be applied by specialized personnel in the different health areas. However, it is considered that training systems for neurological conditions in general can be improved, organized and directed so that the patient learns and participates in a leading role in the course of rehabilitation, with the participation of the family, which can contribute to a rapid improvement.

With the triumph of the Revolution, several studies have been published in Cuban medical journals, among them: Vera Miyar, Morales Pérez (2001); Solís de la Paz, de Armas Casal, García Peñate, Martínez Díaz (2009); Proenza Fernández, Núñez Ramírez, Gallardo Sánchez, de la Paz Castillo (2012).

Our municipality has not lagged behind in the field of research, despite the fact that there are no publications on this subject in Cuban medical journals.

In the analysis of the results during 2013, the following **shortcomings were** detected:

1. Lack of information about the sequelae left by this type of neurological pathology provided to patients, their families and how to educate them to live with them.

2. Failure to use the media to inform and educate the population about this pathology and its rehabilitative treatment.
3. Low motivation of the patient and family towards the rehabilitation process due to lack of knowledge of their pathology.
4. Shortage of technicians in the rehabilitation room to perform land.

Taking into account the insufficiencies found, the following **scientific problem** is posed**:** The lack of knowledge of the patient and the family in rehabilitation does not motivate the systematic participation during therapies. For the solution of the stated problem, the following **objective** is formulated**: To** elaborate a material that gathers information about hemiplegia in ischemic stroke, in order to motivate the patient over 60 years old and his family during the rehabilitation process.

In order to achieve the proposed objectives and to better substantiate and demonstrate the thesis, the following questions and scientific tasks are posed:

Scientific questions

1. What is the historical background underpinning the stroke rehabilitation process?
2. What are the theoretical foundations of the rehabilitation process in hemiplegic patients?
3. What is the current status of stroke in adults (60-74 years old) in the municipality of Guantánamo?
4. What elements are taken into account in the development of information material on stroke rehabilitation?

Scientific Tasks

1. Determination of the historical background of rehabilitation in stroke.
2. Determination of the theoretical foundations that support the rehabilitation process in hemiplegic patients in the municipality of Guantánamo.

3. Characterization of the current state of LCA in the municipality of Guantánamo.
4. Elaboration of a material containing the main information on stroke rehabilitation for patients and their families.

METHODS

Theoretical level:

- **Analysis and synthesis:** to determine the necessary techniques of the theory that supports the dissertation; to elaborate a material, its conclusions and to interpret the diagnosis of the problem.
- **Historical and logical:** to support the historical background of the dissertation and its insertion in the problem at the community level.
- **Induction and deduction:** used in the determination of the rehabilitation treatment to be considered.

Empirical level:

- **Remark:** upon request.
- **Surveys:** to patients with this pathology and their relatives to obtain information about their way of life.
- **Interviews:** to specialists and technicians of the rehabilitation room to diagnose the state of the problem.

Mathematical and statistical level:

- **Percentage analysis:** to process the empirical data obtained and determine the appropriate ratio in the sample.
- **Arithmetic mean:** allows finding the average value around which the data are located.

POPULATION AND SAMPLE

The population explored is made up of 103 patients who attended the rehabilitation room of the Omar Ranedo Pubillones Polyclinic, the sample is made up of 47 patients with a diagnosis of Cerebrovascular Disease, between the ages of 60-74 years, also part of the sample are 100 relatives of patients afflicted by the disease.

CHAPTER I

Historical background underpinning the stroke rehabilitation process

Since ancient times, Hippocrates - recognized as the father of medicine, more than 2,400 years ago - identified and described stroke as "the sudden onset of paralysis".

In ancient times stroke was known as apoplexy*, a general term that physicians applied to anyone suddenly stricken with paralysis. Because many conditions can lead to sudden paralysis, the term stroke did not indicate a specific diagnosis or cause. Physicians knew very little about the cause of the stroke, and the only established therapy was to feed and care for the patient until the stroke ran its course.

The first person to investigate the pathological signs of stroke was Johann Jacob Wepfer. Born in Schaffhausen, Switzerland, in 1620, Wepfer studied medicine and was the first to identify the "postmortem" signs of hemorrhage in the brains of deceased stroke patients. From autopsy studies he gained knowledge about the carotid and vertebral arteries supplying blood to the brain. Wepfer was also the first person to indicate that stroke, in addition to being caused by hemorrhage in the brain, could also be caused by a blockage of one of the main arteries supplying blood to the brain. Thus, stroke came to be known as cerebrovascular disease ("brain" refers to a part of the brain; "vascular" refers to blood vessels and arteries).

Medical science would eventually confirm Wepfer's hypotheses, but until very recently physicians could offer little in the way of therapy. Over the past two decades, basic and clinical researchers, many of them sponsored and funded in part by the National Institute of Neurological Disorders and Stroke (NINDS), have learned a great deal about stroke. (NINDS 2000)

It is true that in Spanish, stroke is popularly known by multiple names: cerebral infarction, thrombosis, embolism, stroke, cerebral hemorrhage, apoplexy, stroke and cerebrovascular disease, which causes great confusion as to the concept and the differentiation between its different types.

Authors define stroke as the result of the occlusion or rupture of a supplementary vessel of the brain. It is the most common of the major central nervous system problems of sudden onset (Matarama, 2005).

Dr. Ruíz García Dania defines stroke as the neurological dysfunction of the Central Nervous System (CNS) due to the affection of the vessels that irrigate it. It is the neurological problem with the greatest epidemiological impact, occupies third place as a cause of death in the western world and generates a notable physical and occupational disability (Authors' Collective, 2002).

Another definition is: Cerebrovascular diseases are the consequence of an alteration of the cerebral circulation that causes a transitory or definitive deficit in the functioning of one or more parts of the brain. We can also define them as all those alterations that affect a part of the brain transiently or permanently by an ischemic or hemorrhagic mechanism. It is an acute neurological dysfunction of vascular origin, of relatively rapid onset, causing focal or sometimes global signs of alteration of brain function lasting more than 24 hours (Collective of authors, 2009).

According to the Spanish Group for the Study of Cerebral Vascular Diseases, stroke is defined as a sudden disturbance of cerebral blood flow that temporarily or permanently alters the function of a specific region of the brain. The term ictus in Spanish is equivalent to "stroke" in English, representing each or all groups of cerebrovascular diseases including cerebral infarction, cerebral hemorrhage or sub-arachnoid hemorrhage (Authors' Collective, 2009).

In the author's opinion, after analyzing the aforementioned concepts, she states: Stroke occurs when the blood supply to a part of the brain is abruptly interrupted or when a blood vessel ruptures, spilling blood into the spaces surrounding the brain cells.

The incidence of stroke increases dramatically with age, the World Health Organization (WHO) considers it the third cause of death and the first cause of disability in the adult world population and it is estimated that 4.5 of the 10 million deaths per year for these reasons belong to non-industrialized countries, a third of the people who survive are left with disabling sequelae and up to 25% of them will present cognitive impairment after the stroke.

Stroke survivors face a variety of mental and physical problems, depending on the severity of the brain damage, but most of them can improve their quality of life through a consistently planned rehabilitation process. In fact, every individual with a condition aspires to rehabilitation, which in many cases is achieved with medical treatment and in others requires specialized technical procedures from other branches of science related to medicine, as is the case of Physiatry.

Rehabilitation through physical exercises are the most frequently used for therapeutic purposes, for the activation of muscular work due to their biological, physiological and psychological significance in the life of man; it helps stroke survivors to reduce their dependence on their caregivers and improve their quality of life. The key to successful rehabilitation includes the attitude of the affected person, the skill of the rehabilitation team, and the social environment (the cooperation of family and friends). (Oraza 2003).

Since the beginning of the revolutionary triumph (1966), Cuban society has dedicated resources and efforts through the Ministry of Public Health to the training of physical therapists. The first steps were taken in hospital institutions such as Frank País, Julio Díaz, Hermanos Almejeiras in the capital and the center for the treatment of neuromotor disorders in Santiago de Cuba.

Cuban teaching programs for residents in the specialty of physical medicine and rehabilitation are nourished (1979) by the collaboration of foreign specialists, such as Dr. Elena Pedraza, a Chilean kinesiologist who contributes to this training (Castro Ruz, 2008).

Cuban doctors Hugo Martínez Sánchez and Eulogio Montoya Guibert began to train the first specialists and the first graduation took place in 1981 at the Julio Díaz Rehabilitation Hospital.

Primary health care rehabilitation services in Cuba are highly developed and are expanding in rural areas, providing coverage to the entire population. In 1984, the family doctor and nurse program was created, which soon incorporated rehabilitation into primary health care.

Cuba is currently making a great effort to improve the quality of life of its population every day. Among the development programs carried out by Cuban public health is the creation of multiple Integral Rehabilitation rooms in Primary Health Care, equipped with the highest and most modern technology. This new service interrelates a group of specialties such as: Defectology, Speech Therapy, Psychology, Occupational Therapy, Podiatry, Physical Therapy and Rehabilitation, all working in an integral way, applying treatments for the prevention and care of diseases, constituting physical therapy and rehabilitation one of the specialties of greater weight in the effective and rapid recovery of the patient.

These services rehabilitate patients with various pathologies, among which neurological conditions stand out, including stroke, which is the third leading cause of death in the developed world, after cardiovascular diseases and cancer, as well as the leading cause of disability in the elderly, due to the motor, sensory and cognitive sequelae in most of the patients who survive this disease.

In the province of Guantánamo, the development of rehabilitation at the primary care level began with the creation of the first room in the main municipality, belonging to the central area, on July 23, 2004, which was inaugurated with four technicians and Dr. Santiago Almenares as specialist. Today, with the development of this process, these figures have increased and there is a rehabilitation room for each municipality and popular councils, which has a specialist or a diploma holder, and a greater number of technicians.

Theoretical foundations of the rehabilitation process in hemiplegic patients.

Cerebrovascular disease is a health problem with a high social and economic impact, because it affects a large number of functionally and occupationally active people, generates disabilities and sequelae and has high costs for the health system. (Coll Costa, 2008)

The rehabilitation process in Cuba is structured on the basis of the most advanced of contemporary science and in total correspondence with the Marxist-Leninist ideology. The scientific character implies taking sides with scientific truth and its humanistic use in response to this ideology (Castro Ruz, 2008).

Psychological:

Survivors of a stroke must face a variety of mental and physical problems, the sequelae always involve a certain degree of dependence and loss of autonomy among adults, causing damage to activities of daily living such as feeding, dressing, personal hygiene care, use of household appliances, use of transportation, among others, these limitations bring with them isolation, depression, anxiety, being a carrier of physical disability compromises the person and the environment, especially the family. Emotional and affective support must be present throughout the development of rehabilitation, which will enable an active and interested participation in the process, which significantly influences the development of their activity.

Social:

It is a social challenge because about 30% to 40% of survivors in the first year after the stroke are not able to return to work and require some kind of help to perform basic activities of daily living, thus society loses people useful for its development. Rehabilitation is based on working on labor reinsertion.

Economic:

The treatment of this disease is very costly for the country because the patient requires admission to a hospital institution and frequent attendance to the rehabilitation room.

On the other hand, for the family it also has an economic impact, as the patient needs to be transferred to receive consultations and therapies for a speedy recovery.

Role of health personnel:

It constitutes a serious problem because the therapies are prolonged and the patient becomes upset.

There should be a process of collaboration between the patient, family and health professionals during the rehabilitation period. This collaboration is not limited to the hospital environment and should continue throughout the course of the disease.

In the special conditions in which the family and patients suffering from this neurological condition find themselves, it is necessary to educate them in the prevention and control of risk factors.

Develop health actions aimed at raising awareness among stroke patients about the importance of attending therapies.

The principle of linkage with life, work and the practice of communist construction. Modifying personality traits in these patients is closely linked to the concept of rehabilitation, which implies their insertion in the social environment, in its various manifestations such as study, work, recreation, among others.

This principle is present from the planning of the different activities that are developed during rehabilitation, in which the barriers between the institution and social life are broken down, making them respond to social needs, allowing each patient to have an active participation in their transformation, expanding their experiences in the different social tasks, in their new conditions, including working conditions, taking into account their individual particularities, interests and motivations.

Patients are educated to be able to coexist in society, in a dignified manner, as useful individuals, joining labor and social activities, without constituting a social burden, which ratifies the humanistic character of the Cuban revolution (Llanes Torres, Alonso Pavón, Amaro Hernández, 2010).

The rehabilitation process for patients with neurological diseases takes place within the framework of a group of people, who are grouped according to different criteria, with certain characteristics. Each member has unique characteristics that distinguish him/her from the rest, who have the right to be respected and considered, acquiring relevant importance the knowledge of the problems, needs and professional and individual interests of the patients, which allows guiding and teaching them to choose the best alternative and stimulate their results.

In this process, all actions foresee working in favor of the patient, taking into account his or her needs, interests and characteristics; as well as increasing the use of independent work methods so that the level of demand is progressively raised, based on self-learning and self-control, where the family plays an important role.

Emotional and affective support is present throughout the rehabilitation process, which enables an active and interested participation in the process, which significantly influences the development of their activity.

In rehabilitation, it is essential to assess and reconcile the process to the individual particularities (age, school level, personal background, stage of the disease, time of suffering, among others). Its concretion is possible from the organization, planning and management of the rehabilitation task, which are developed in consideration of the characteristics of the group and the patient.

Based on this consideration, the following are determined: the content, forms, methods and means to direct the process, taking into account within the group the disabilities of each patient and their real possibilities, for which the objectives to be followed in each patient must be adapted.

In the conditions of the work we carry out, the objective reality posed to the family is of vital importance, in the material conditions of the home, for each of the members, the living conditions, the economic and social activity of its members and in particular those presented to patients with neurological conditions, which has an important subjective repercussion.

Scientific studies carried out in the country on the way of life of the Cuban family (ICCP-2001) show, among other factors, those that influence the emotional state of each of the members of the family.

Another important element about the family is to consider it not only as a simple cell that makes up the social fabric and depends on historical or cultural forces, but also as a unit where its members understand and share interests, feelings and emotional relationships whose psychological climate has an impact on the activity of its members (Castro Alegret, 2004).

In the special conditions in which the family and the patients suffering from this neurological condition find themselves, it is necessary to take members, the ways for their preparation in order to allow their active and systematic participation in the rehabilitation process during the sessions directed by the rehabilitator, to give them continuity at home and to achieve their active incorporation in the family and social bosom in dignified coexistence with the effects of the disease they suffer from.

This communication is essential to achieve the success of the rehabilitation treatment; so that the patient accepts his illness and the direct attention to his major difficulties and concerns, the clarification of the ways through which his recovery should be carried out, the adequate selection and dosage of the objectives in each task and the objective evaluation of his achievements and failures, stimulates him to integrate himself to the development of the rehabilitation.

To the extent that the hemiplegic patient has greater autonomy and independence, his or her emotional state is also favored, which allows the satisfaction of being able to help at home and thus improve the patients' perception of family relationships (Gómez Juanola, Machín Díaz, Roque Acanda, Hernández Medina, 2001).

It is also known that united families, with a tendency towards harmony, balance and positive interactions, show better adaptive capacities that predict success in facing existential frustrations, as well as creative family restructuring in the face of events that generate suffering.

Quality of life as a measure of the impact of a disease on an individual has a predictive value for physical function and well-being, in addition to the fact that hemiplegia has an impact on physical functioning; this is the most affected dimension, but the final result will depend on the ability to adapt to the new life situation and this will be better to the extent that better treatments are implemented. Anxiety and depression were the most evident psychological symptoms in these patients (Suárez Escudero, Restrepo Cano, Ramírez, Liliana Bedoya, 2011).

Characterization of the current state of LCA in the municipality of Guantánamo.

Knowing the state of health of the population as well as its demands has always been an object of concern of the Cuban state, which has materialized in different actions, programs and levels of care, such as primary health care, where family doctors and nurses play an important role, who are in charge of dispensing geriatric patients in order to provide them with special care and contribute to guaranteeing them not only a longer, but also a more active and healthy life. Nowadays, when the elderly population in Cuba exceeds one and a half million inhabitants, the health sector and other sectors, institutions and government demand the periodic updating of indicators that trace their health conditions in order to privilege this vulnerable group of the population.

The **incidence of** the Omar Ranedo pubillones polyclinic during the year 2023, there was a total of 103 patients of both sexes, who have suffered a stroke, which represents 100%, and this shows me the increase that has existed over the years, and could be due to the fact that Cuba is in the fourth and final phase of the demographic transition, with very low levels of fertility and mortality and although it is not the most aged country in Latin America, it will be in a few years, as a consequence of its social development and the advanced stage of its demographic transition, there is an increase in the risk factors that favor the appearance of neurological diseases.

In order to know the current state of the problem under investigation, different instruments were applied: interviews to specialists, technicians, and surveys to patients and family members.

The research instruments applied were the following.

- **Remark:** upon request.
- **Surveys:** to patients with this pathology and their relatives to obtain information about their way of life.
- **Interviews:** to specialists and technicians of the rehabilitation room.

Observation was used to discover the phenomena that arise in the performance of specialists in directing the rehabilitation of patients, the interview was used to collect information about the rehabilitation of these patients with ischemic stroke and their families, as well as their results for the design of the rehabilitation process based on the transformation and protagonism of the patient, the survey allowed to know the level of mastery of the basic contents of the patient and his family about the disease. (See Annexes 1 and 2). It was found that some family members of patients affected by ischemic stroke in the study population do not attend therapies with them, do not provide them with the emotional support necessary for their recovery, and render them useless at home, so that they do not allow them to perform some activities of daily living (ADLs).

When interpreting the surveys applied to the 47 patients, 16 patients answered that their relatives always accompany them to the therapies, which represents 34.0%, 18 answered sometimes, representing 38.2% and 13 answered never, representing 27.6%, which shows me that most of the relatives of these patients do not support them emotionally, for their prompt recovery.

When the survey was applied to the 100 relatives, they answered in the questions about how the family applied some rehabilitative treatment at home to their relative, 32 responded that always, which represents 32%, 36 relatives responded that sometimes in the evenings because work did not allow them to waste time since that corresponds to the rehabilitation room, representing 36%, and the rest (32) responded that never, because that is why the patient went to the rehabilitation room, representing 32%. In the other question where: Do you think you would improve if you as a family helped him in his rehabilitation treatment: 32 family members answered yes, representing 32%, and 68 family members answered no, that if their family member does not improve it is because the treatment was not the best, and that is the fault of the doctor and the technician of the rehabilitation room, representing 68% of the sample.

From the interviews conducted with the physicians and technicians who work in the rehabilitation room, they indicate coincidence in terms of the criteria expressed: that patients who come to the room in some cases is the first time they attend the consultation, and present ignorance of the importance of this medical specialty for their recovery due to the sequelae left by their disease (stroke); some patients arrive at the stage of spasticity which their recovery is slow unlike other patients who come to the room immediately after discharge from the hospital, several patients abandon the treatment because it is long term; The relatives of the affected patients do not accompany them to the therapies, so the disabled patient feels depressed and is unable to attend the therapies, which influences their mood and their physical, psychological and social recovery.

Application of the educational intervention for the stroke patient over 60 years of age.

It is a proposal that is aimed at providing the patient with an orientation guide for the application of a correct rehabilitation, since it offers exercise alternatives that the patient can choose to modify his or her lifestyle.

This intervention is based on the analysis of the practical experience we have developed in our professional work, in addition to a critical bibliographic study of the programs related to rehabilitation. Its application in practice, prepares the patient who has suffered a Cerebrovascular Accident for its correct rehabilitation.

The objectives of the rehabilitative treatment that the physiatrist is going to draw before a hemiplegic patient should be:

- Psychological support.
- Prevent complications.
- Achieving independence in the A.V.D.'s.
- Increase muscle power and dexterity on the affected side and preserve the healthy side.
- Improve coordination and balance.
- To achieve the most functional and aesthetic gait possible.
- Improve communication disorder.
- Work on labor reinsertion.

For the elaboration of this informative material where the most important aspects of this pathology and the sequelae that the patient presents afterwards are collected, we must know that hemiplegia is one of them, and the one that most limits the patient in his social performance and influences his psychic and emotional state.

Hemiplegia is characterized by the loss of voluntary movements in one half of the body together with the alteration of postural tone that may be increased (spasticity), decreased (flaccidity) or both elements at the same time" (Alonso López, Pérez Sánchez, Peñate Recio, 2001).

The sample was selected by the patients of the rehabilitation room of the Omar Ranedo Pubillones Polyclinic, it is composed of 47 patients with the pathology of Cerebrovascular Disease of Ischemic type, and that have as sequel a hemiplegia, between the ages of 60-74 years, constituting the population, which represents 100%, also part of the sample 100 relatives of patients afflicted by the disease.

Of the total number of patients: 31 men (65.9%) and 16 women (34.0%) (see Table 1), it can be seen how many patients were treated for ischemic CVD by the Rehabilitation Service during the period studied. There was a predominance of the male sex for 65.9%, which reaffirms the theory of the protection produced by female hormones in the adult stage of women.

Table 2 shows the distribution by age and sex, which shows that in the male sex between the ages of 64 and 66 years there are a total of 5 patients, representing 10.6% of the population under study.In the female sex there is a predominance in the ages of 64 and 73 years with 3 patients, representing 6.4%; the most predominant age when adding both sexes is 64 years with 8 patients, which means (17%) of 100%, followed by the age of 66 years with 5 patients, representing (10.6%) of the population studied.

From neurological physiotherapy, cognitive and sensory stimulation to gait re-education and progressive recovery of autonomy in the development of daily activities.

The treatments to which patients will be submitted will also be determined according to the phase of the disease in which they are. In the acute phase, the important thing will be to focus on the prevention of complications, postural treatment and patient independence. In the subacute and chronic phase, recovering balance and gait and resorting to kinesitherapy and maintenance physiotherapy, all these activities are aimed at helping the patient regain his or her independence to carry out daily tasks.

Despite the fact that the therapeutic benefit decreases with the age of the patient, several studies have shown that the degree of disability presented by elderly patients on admission can be significantly reduced after undergoing rehabilitation treatment. And that is why it is essential that the elderly have access to them, without being limited by age.

Some people are subject to a higher risk of suffering a stroke than others. For better study we will divide the risk factors into:

Non Modifiable:

- Age.
- Family history.
- Sex.
- Race.

Modifiable by treatment:

- Arterial hypertension.
- Heart disease.
- Diabetes mellitus.
- Previous stroke.
- Carotid stenosis.

Modifiable by behavior:

- Hypercholesterolemia.
- Sedentary lifestyle.
- Drug addiction.
- Smoking.
- Alcoholism.
- Obesity.

Non-modifiable risk factors

Older people have a higher risk of suffering a stroke than the general population; for every decade after the age of 60, the risk of this disease doubles.

The gender or sex of the person also contributes as a risk factor for suffering a stroke. Men have a 1.25 times higher risk of suffering this pathology than women.

Risk factors modifiable by treatment

There are many diseases that can trigger a stroke, among those mentioned:

Arterial Hypertension

Of all the factors, the most important is that people with hypertension have a risk four to six times higher than those who do not suffer from this disease. From 40 to 90% of people are found to have high blood pressure (BP) before the stroke occurs. Antihypertensive medication can reduce the risk of this disease. Recent studies indicate that treatment can reduce the incidence rate of stroke by 38% and reduce the mortality rate by 40%.

Heart disease

After hypertension, it is the second most important risk factor, among them can be found: malformations of the heart valves or heart muscle. Some valvular diseases such as mitral valve stenosis or mitral annular calcification can double the risk of stroke, independently of other risk factors.

Diabetes Mellitus

This disease reaches the highest point of risk between the ages of 50 and 60 years and decreases after these ages, is higher in men at an earlier age and higher in women at an older age. People with diabetes may also have other factors that can contribute to an increased overall risk of stroke.

Behaviorally modifiable risk factors

Hypercholesterolemia

High cholesterol levels contribute to heart disease. But many people do not understand that high cholesterol also contributes to stroke risk. Foods high in saturated fat and cholesterol, such as meats, eggs and dairy products, can increase the amount of total cholesterol in the body to alarming levels, contributing to the risk of atherosclerosis.

Smoking

It is the most powerful modifiable risk factor contributing to cerebrovascular disease. Cigarette smoking almost doubles a person's risk of ischemic stroke, independent of other factors, heavy smokers are subject to a higher risk of stroke than less regular smokers. This risk decreases immediately after quitting smoking, with a significant reduction in risk observed after 2 to 4 years. Unfortunately, it may take several decades for an ex-smoker's risk to drop to the level of a person who has never smoked.

Alcoholism

An increase in alcohol consumption leads to an increase in blood pressure and ischemic stroke.

Drug addiction

The use of illicit drugs, such as cocaine and crack cocaine, can also cause stroke. Cocaine can act on other risk factors, such as hypertension and heart disease, triggering a stroke.

Marijuana use is also a risk factor, it lowers blood pressure and can interact with other factors, such as hypertension and cigarette smoking, causing damage to blood vessels.

Other drugs of abuse, such as amphetamines, heroin and anabolic steroids (and even some common legal drugs, such as caffeine and the Lasparaginase and pseudoephedrine found in over-the-counter decongestants), have been suspected of increasing a person's risk of stroke. Many of these drugs are vasoconstrictors, which means they can cause blood vessels to constrict and increase blood pressure.

When analyzing the risk factors with respect to the total population studied, we can analyze (see Table 5) that there is a predominance of occasional drinkers, with the total male population being 31, representing 66% of the total sample (47), followed by 24 hypertensive patients, representing 51%, and 22 sedentary patients, representing 47%; with respect to the female population, arterial hypertension predominates with 13 patients, corresponding to 28% of the population studied, followed by 12 patients with Diabetes Mellitus, representing 25.5%.

We can analyze that in the female population there is a lower number of sedentary patients, and this may be due to the fact that the rest of the population (7) is linked to the grandparents' circles of the community to which they belong.

Stroke rehabilitation is a program that encompasses different therapies designed to help you relearn skills lost after a stroke. Depending on the area affected by the stroke, rehabilitation can help you regain movement, speech, strength and daily living skills. Stroke rehabilitation can help you regain independence and improve your quality of life.

The complications of stroke vary widely, as does how each person recovers afterwards. Studies have shown that people who participate in a specialized stroke rehabilitation program do better than most people who do not do rehabilitation. Consequently, rehabilitation is recommended for all people who have had a stroke. Rehabilitation treatment will depend on the stage of the disease at which the patient has reached, and the time in which it starts, it should begin 24-48h, after recovery, is based primarily on: reintegrate the patient as far as possible in his previous life, prepare him psychologically giving him confidence and development, interconsultations at home and work in the gym depending on the hemiplegia.

The recovery of a patient can be stopped at any of the stages of the disease, if treatment cannot be done immediately after the hemiplegia is installed, it must be started at the stage at which the patient has arrived, which are:

1. Initial stage of flaccidity.
2. Spasticity stage.
3. Relative recovery stage.

It should be kept in mind that the stages overlap and cannot be neatly separated. Certain degrees of spasticity may already be present during the flaccid stage, or the patient may have some fairly independent limb movement during the spastic stage. Furthermore, even in the third stage, spasticity may still hinder selective movements when the patient struggles to perform a difficult task.

Initial stage of flaccidity

This stage is observed soon after the hemiplegia is established, lasting from a few days to several weeks or more. The patient cannot move the affected hemibody. He has lost contact with the diseased side and often does not feel the respective arm or leg. Therefore, **proprioceptive and sensory stimulation of the healthy side** will be used: the healthy foot will move over the whole of the paralyzed lower limb and the upper limb will move over the affected side, this will help to improve or anticipate the alterations of the body scheme.

The patient adopts a position in bed where the affected side appears to be slightly rotated slightly backwards, usually the patient cannot turn to the healthy side. He/she does not sit up if not supported and tends to fall towards the ill side.

Postural treatment

At this stage, collaboration with the nursing staff or family members is of paramount importance, because the patient's position in bed must be monitored, changing it frequently, this will be maintained 24 hours a day, every 2 hours, to prevent complications such as: tendinomuscular retractions, avoid ulcers and pathological postures, and infections. The bed will be of rigid frame and soft mattress, the sheets will be clean, stretched and at adequate temperature.

- Supine decubitus: Patient with good alignment in bed, pillows on the head, under the shoulder and affected hip, and small roller on the affected hand and popliteal fossa on the same side, feet at a 90 degree angle supported to the bedside to avoid equinus.
- Prone decubitus: When pulmonary, cardiovascular and skeletal status permit, this position is advantageous for the maintenance of full extension of the hips and relief of pressure on the bony eminences. Patient well aligned, large pillow under the shoulder and affected arm, and medium pillow under the abdomen, and rollers under the patella and anterior area of the ankle joint and on the affected hand, feet resting on the skin at an angle of 90 degrees.
- Lateral Decubitus: Hemiplegics are most comfortable on the sound side, never lying on the affected side. A large pillow will be placed supporting the affected upper limb with the elbow in flexion and roller in the hand, and another large pillow under the affected lower limb with the knee in 90 degree flexion, as well as the feet.

Development of sitting balance

The patient should be seated as early as possible, in the first 48-72 hours, first in bed and then out of bed, with the feet resting on the floor, protecting the upper extremity with a sling while it is flaccid. Insist from the beginning on trying to achieve good balance by performing balance exercises in this position.

At this stage, the hemiplegic patient often stumbles with difficulty looking up from a sitting position, because he tends to fall backwards when he raises his head and extends his spine.

The physical therapist remains in front of him and encourages him to move his body forward, flexing the hip joints as much as possible, while raising his arms and placing his hands on his (the therapist's) shoulders. When he is able to maintain this position and has the spine well extended, he induces him to lift his chin and look upwards. This counteracts the tendency to fall backwards by giving the patient sufficient flexion at the hips.

Spasticity stage

At this stage, spasticity usually develops slowly, with a predilection for the flexor muscles of the arm and the extensor muscles of the lower limb. As spasticity develops, resistance is registered for certain passive movements, passive mobilizations of the affected hemibody and instruction of self-passive mobilization, performed by the patient himself with the help of the healthy side, will be performed.

Passive movement awareness

Under verbal commands; achieving a control of the affected side and the healthy side where the patient recognizes the position of the different structures of his body. The patient should not go on to perform more complex movements but to overcome or learn the previous simpler ones.

When seated, he leans more on the healthy side than on the diseased side. The affected arm is in flexion, with the spastic leg in greater abduction than the healthy one. At this stage the patient is able to stand, but rests almost all of his weight on the sound leg. He has usually learned to walk abnormally.

Development of balance in standing

The patient begins to sit and stand up with assistance at the beginning, then without using the hands and in the most symmetrical and normal way possible using the tilt table. Once a standing position in front of the mirror is achieved, the postural reeducation will be done, then we will start with balance exercises in this position in order to prepare the patient to start the gait reeducation (Coll Costa, 2008).

Phase I:

- Tilting table

- Progressive bipedestation between parallels. (A posture in front of the mirror will be performed, a step will not be taken until the static posture is good.
- Balance.
- Pace restart patterns (Static patterns)

Phase II:

- Dynamic patterns in parallel.
- Parallel coordination patterns.
- Correction of alterations in the gait phase.
- Auxiliary support training.
- Postural correction during ambulation.

Phase III:

- Dynamic patterns out of parallels.
- Dynamic patterns on smooth and uneven terrain.
- Patterns with change of rhythm and direction.
- Correction of coordination between auxiliary support and support balance.

Phase IV:

- Dynamic walking patterns on all types of terrain.
- Going up and down stairs and inclined planes.
- Training in falls and incorporations.

Stimulation of active contractions

Perform 4 to 6 repetitions per day, very short to avoid fatigue, selectively and progressively. Upper limb in shoulder abduction and elbow flexion. Lower limb in plantar extension of the foot and hip and knee flexion aided by manual resistance. Direct muscle stimulation with stretching, kneading and tapping.

In gait, the patient tends to keep the whole of the diseased side slightly backward. It seems as if he is dragging it with the healthy side. He does not rotate the shoulder girdle or swing his arms. A more normal gait pattern is obtained by employing trunk rotation as follows. The technician stands in front of the patient, holding both hands. As the patient steps with the right foot, say, the kinesiologist swings both arms diagonally to the right, with the left arm forward and the right arm slightly backward, rotating the patient's shoulder girdle.

As the patient transfers weight forward on the right leg and steps forward with the left leg, the kinesiologist reverses the arm motion. Rhythmic arm swing and trunk rotation contribute to the development of a normal bilateral gait pattern. The arm movements must be well synchronized to match the patient's steps.

Progression of active contraction (TFNP)

By increasing contractile activity agonist and antagonist muscles should progress in parallel, an automatism will be achieved through the patient's attention, executing movements with accuracy and coordination, as well as their repetition and increase of executions, e.g. eating, writing, being of help occupational therapy.

Resistance is used to facilitate the muscle's ability to contract, increases muscle control, helps the patient gain an awareness of movement and its direction, and increases strength.

Manual contact makes pressure on the muscle helps the muscle's ability to contract.

The traction and approximation makes the movement easier, especially in traction movements and antigravitational movements.

Aids in the elongation of muscle tissue when the stretch reflex is used.

Stretching facilitates muscle contraction. Verbal stimulation is carried out by verbally telling the patient what to do and when to do it.

The use of vision helps the patient to control and correct his or her position and movement.

Specific techniques

1. Rhythmic initiation: It is the rhythmic movement of the limb or body through the desired path, starting with passive movement and progressing to active resisted movement. With the aim that the subject is able to: initiate the movement, improve coordination and sense of movement, normalize the speed of movement, increase or decrease it, teach the movement, this technique helps the patient to relax.
2. Slow inversion: Active movement changes from one direction (Agonist) to the opposite (Antagonist) without pause or relaxation. In order to: increase joint amplitude, endurance and strength, develop coordination, prevent or reduce fatigue.
3. Rhythmic stabilization: Alternate isometric contractions against resistance, no intention of movement. Aiming to: increase strength, stability, balance and decrease pain.

Treatment

It is the continuation of the first stage, here a more advanced unfolding of the total modalities is initiated, in order to obtain a more appropriate adaptation of the movements to the functional activities in the different positions.

Active or active resisted movements will be made progressively and the patient will collaborate in transfers from chair to bed, from bed to chair, toileting, feeding and changing clothes.

Relative recovery stage

Some patients recover so well that they are able to use their hand quite well and their gait is almost normal. At this stage spasticity is always mild. However, certain small localized movements of the elbow, wrist and fingers, as well as of the knee, ankle and fingers, cannot be performed. The limbs still move too much as a whole, and intrinsic movements are missing. Therefore, treatment is oriented towards obtaining even more localized, finer and more isolated movements. For this purpose, the reflex inhibitory modalities are even further unfolded. The physiotherapist prevents movements in the neighboring joints when the patient moves his wrist or fingers.

Occupational therapy

- Sensory-motor attention.
- Independence activities for ADLs.
- Professional recovery.
- Adaptation to daily activities.
- Manual dominance skills.
- Need of auxiliary means for its performance.
- Coordination, manual dexterity and processing activities.

Speech therapy

Based on capacities of: memory, coordination of movements through specialized movements, mastery of articulation, intelligence, attention, emotions and previous communication experiences.

Vocational guidance and employment

Within the rehabilitation process we must take into account the patient's professional training to establish the vocational prognosis, which will be determined by:

- The physical ability or activity that the patient can perform despite residual disability.
- Mental abilities and intelligence.

- Previous work history.
- Personality and social adaptation.
- Economic possibilities.

What we have just formulated of the treatment of the hemiplegic patient is only an outline, the way to proceed with the patient cannot be described in more detail because the physical therapist will have to develop his own technique and continually adjust his handling of the patient according to the patient's reactions. He will have to wait for the patient's response when placing him in a position or moving him, and his next therapeutic step will depend on what he considers or observes. By inhibiting abnormal reactions and facilitating more normal reactions whenever you can, the patient will gradually acquire more motor responses to your handling. Eventually he will learn to develop the same movement modalities actively and without assistance.

By applying this treatment to the population studied, we can see that the improvement of the hemiplegic patient will not depend exclusively on the rehabilitation treatment, but on the stage at which the therapies are initiated after the stroke, and on family support, which affects the emotional state, and on the disposition of each family during the treatment.

In the sample studied, 47 patients attended the rehabilitation room after discharge from the hospital, to begin therapies, of them: 16 patients their relative took them to the room to perform the exercise sessions, and at home they performed some of them, representing 34.0%, 18 relatives took the patient to the room leaving them at the center, and returned after the therapies were concluded, and sometimes they did not take them, and neither did they help them at home representing 38.2%, and the rest of the patients (13) their relatives took them to the therapies when they could, they did not assist them with the exercises at home, representing 27.7%.

At the end of 2023, 16 patients who had suffered an ischemic stroke were discharged from the rehabilitation room. They were rehabilitated and included in the grandparents' circle of their community, and were assigned home activities to stimulate their emotional state, so that they would feel useful and independent in society, unlike the rest of the patients, who had insufficient support and attention from their families, although they were satisfied with the care provided by the physiatrist and the technician who attended them.

Cuba is a socialist country where medical assistance is free and care is provided to any individual who needs it. We must keep in mind that the family is the fundamental cell of society, where each person finds love and comfort in the face of illness, and influences the rapid recovery of each of its members.

CONCLUSIONS

- Knowledge of the history of this branch of medicine helps to improve the general and integral culture of the population.
- It was demonstrated that there was a lack of knowledge on the part of patients and their families about the management of rehabilitation treatment in this pathology.
- The material presented shows that not only the rehabilitative treatment influences the rapid recovery of the patient, but also the psychological support of the family plays an important role.

REFERENCES BIBLIOGRAPHIC REFERENCES

Alonso López, R. F., Pérez Sánchez, A., Peñate Recio, P. O. (2001). Utility of synkinetic physical exercise in motor reeducation of the neurotransplanted hemiplegic. *Efdeportes*, *7*(38).

Alvarez Sintes, R., Hernández Cabrera, G., Báster Moro, J. C., García Núñez, R. D., Louro Bernal, I., Céspedes Lantigua, L. A. (2008). *Comprehensive general medicine*. Havana: Editorial Ciencias Médicas, 1, 278.

Caballero López, A. D. (2008). *Terapia Intensiva*. Editorial Ciencias Médicas. Havana Volume III.

Cárdenas de la Peña, E. (2004) *Medical Terminology*. McGraw-Hill. Interamericana. Third edition.

Castro Alegret, P. L. (2004) *The teacher and the family of the adult with difficulties*. ICCP

Castro, F. (2008). *Reflections of the commander in chief*. Government of Reconciliation and National Unity.

Authors' collective (2009). *Rehabilitation of adults with cerebral vascular disease*. Mexico: Secretaría de Salud.

Collective of authors (2002). *Manual de diagnóstico y tratamiento en especialidades clínicas*. Editora Política, Havana,

Collective of authors (2005). *Merk's manual of diagnosis and treatment*. Staff Publishing House. London,

Collective of authors. (2009) *Comprehensive management of cerebrovascular diseases in primary health care*.

Coll Costa, J. L. (2008). *Rehabilitation of hemiplegic patients*. https://www.guiadisc.com/wp-content/uploads/2012/12/rehabilitacion-hemiplejicos.pdf

Larousse Illustrated Dictionary (1988). Editorial Pueblo y Educación. Havana,

Editorial Científico Técnica (1998) *Terminological dictionary of medical sciences.* 11 E. Havana

Estévez Perera, A., Coll Costa, J. D. L., Estévez Perera, A. (2011). Satisfaction of hemiplegic patients after an individualized physical exercise program. *Cuban Journal of General Comprehensive Medicine*, *27*(1), 74-82. http://scielo.sld.cu/scielo.php?pid=S0864-21252011000100008&script=sci_arttext

Farreras, P., Rozman, C. (2005). *Medicina interna* 14 ed. Editorial Elsevier, 108-116.

Fernández Nieves, Y., López Bueno, M., Barrios González, J. E., Coll Costa, J. (2008) Disability and attention to diversity: a challenge to science. *EFDeportes.com, Digital Magazine*. Buenos Aires, Nº 123. http://www.efdeportes.com/efd123/discapacidad-y-atencion-a-la-diversidad-un-desafio-a-la-ciencia.htm

Gómez Juanola, M., Machín Díaz, M. J., Roque Acanda, K., Hernández Medina, G. (2001). Considerations about the geriatric patient. *Revista cubana de medicina general integral*, *17*(5), 468-472. http://scielo.sld.cu/scielo.php?pid=S0864-21252001000500010&script=sci_arttext

González, M. R., Kindelán Alosnso, B. (1997). Physiotherapy of hemiplegia*, in su: Medical Rehabilitation*. Editorial MASSON, Chap. 11, p 131-143.

Knott, M., Voss, D. E. (1974). *Proprioceptive neuromuscular facilitation: patterns and techniques*. Editorial medica panamericana.

Llanes Torres, H. M., Alonso Pavón, Y., Amaro Hernández, A. H. (2010) Behavior of mortality due to cerebrovascular disease in the municipality of Madruga. *Medimay*, *16*(1), 13-19. https://scholar.archive.org/work/lsponbrxlvernc25yu7nz22s2i/access/way

back/http://www.medimay.sld.cu/index.php/rcmh/article/download/450/773

Llanio Navarro, R., Perdomo González, G. (2003). *Propedéutica clínica y semiología médica v1.* Ciencias Médicas. https://apunteca.usal.edu.ar/id/eprint/1191/28/Cap.27%20Alteraciones%20de%20la%20temperatura%20corporal.pdf

Matarama Peñate, M. (2005) *Medicina Interna. Diagnosis and treatment*. Havana: Editorial Ciencias Médicas.

Maya, C. (2007). *Neurological emergencies*. Editorial Ciencias Médicas.

Melgar, F., Penny, E. (2012). *Geriatrics and gerontology for the internist*. La Paz: Grupo Editorial La Hoguera.

Ministry of Public Health (May 20, 2015) Official Gazette No. 17 Extraordinary. https://www.cecmed.cu/sites/default/files/adjuntos/Reglamentacion/Resoluci%C3%B3n%20MINSAP%20381-%202015.pdf

Ministry of Public Health [MINSAP] (1992) Objectives, purposes and guidelines to increase the health of the Cuban population 1992-2000. Havana: Editorial Ciencias Médicas

Ministry of Public Health [MINSAP] (2022) Anuario estadístico de salud. National Directorate of Medical Records and Health Statistics. Havana. Cuba. 22 http://files.sld.cu/bvscuba/files/2012/05/anuario-2021-e.pdf

National Institute of Neurological Disorders and Stroke [NINDS] (2000). Stroke*: Hope in research.* http://espanol.ninds.nih.gov/trastrornos/accidente_cerebrovascular.htm

World Health Organization (WHO). (1979). *Optimal adult physical performance capacity*. Technical Information Series. WHO

Orosa Fraiz, T. (2003). La tercera edad y la familia, una mirada desde el adulto mayor. *Havana: Editorial Félix Varela*, 67-93.

Proenza Fernández, L., Núñez Ramírez, L., Gallardo Sánchez, Y., & de la Paz Castillo, K. L. (2012). Knowledge and lifestyle modification in older adults with cerebrovascular disease. *Medisan*, *16*(10), 1540-1547. http://scielo.sld.cu/scielo.php?pid=S1029-30192012001000009&script=sci_arttext

Roca Goderich, R. (2002) *Temas de Medicina Interna (*Volume I). Editorial Ciencias Médicas. 4th Edition.

Rodríguez Silva, H. M., Pérez Caballero, M. D. (2002). Manual de Diagnóstico y tratamiento en especialidades clínicas. *Havana: Editora Política*, 205-7.

Solís de la Paz, D., de Armas Casal, D. L., García Peñate, G., & Martínez Díaz, N. (2009). Influence of prognostic factors in the recovery of patients with cerebrovascular disease. *Habanera Journal of Medical Sciences*, *8*(1), http://scielo.sld.cu/scielo.php?pid=S1729-519X2009000100007&script=sci_arttext

Suárez Escudero, J. C., Restrepo Cano, S. C., Ramírez, E. P., Liliana Bedoya, C. (2011). Clinical, social, occupational and individual functional perception description in stroke patients. *Acta Neurológica Colombiana*, *27*(2), 97-105. http://www.scielo.org.co/scielo.php?pid=S0120-87482011000200003&script=sci_arttext

Torres Carro, O. (2008). *Pedagogical strategy for neurological rehabilitation, 120h* [Thesis in option to the scientific degree of Doctor in Pedagogical Sciences. Central Institute of Pedagogical Sciences. Havana]. https://tesis.sld.cu/index.php?P=DownloadFile&Id=597

Vera Miyar, C. R., & Morales Pérez, C. (2001). Cerebrovascular disease: follow-up and rehabilitation in the community. *Revista Cubana de Medicina General Integral*, *17*(1), 27-34. http://scielo.sld.cu/scielo.php?pid=S0864-21252001000100004&script=sci_arttext&tlng=en

Zorowitz, R. D. (1997). Rehabilitation of the patient with cerebral vascular accident. *González Mas R. Medical rehabilitation. Barcelona: Masson*, 432-560.

ANNEXES

Annex 1

Stroke Patient Survey

Age ________ Sex __________

Time since stroke ______________________________

Type of sequel left: Sequel _______ No sequel ______

Current treatment: Temporary _______ Permanent ______

Personal pathological history:

HTN ______ Smoking ________ Diabetes ________ Heart disease ______ Obesity ______ Alcohol intake ___________ Other ______

Time taken to hospital:

Less than 2 h _______ 2 to 5 h ______ more than 6 h _______

Time in which physiotherapy began:

Immediate ______ Medium ______ Late ______ Never _____

Capacity for independence:

I- Eat

Without assistance ______ With assistance _______ Needs to be fed _______

II- Washing

Without assistance _______ With assistance _______

III- Body care (hairstyle, brushing, shaving)

Without assistance ______ With assistance ______

IV- Dressing

No help ____ With help ____Only with possible help ____Completely unable ____

V- From a bed to a wheelchair

Unassisted use of wheelchair _______

Requires some assistance ________

Can sit up, but needs constant assistance ______

Permanent in bed _______

VI- Movement capacity

Can walk 50 steps (with cane, without walker) ______ in a wheelchair _______con helps__________

VII- Stair climbing

Without outside help ______Only with help _______Impossible ______

VIII- Your family member attends therapy with you.

Yes____ No____ Sometimes_____.

Annex 2

Survey for the family with a family member who is hemiplegic due to a stroke.

Mark with an X as appropriate.

Questions:

1- You know your family member's illness:

Yes _____ No _____

2- Do you know which are the modifiable risk factors that your family member has?:_____________

3- Allows you to make decisions as a member of the household despite your illness:

Always _____ Sometimes _____ Never_____

4- Your family's disability causes you to be limited in activities of daily living.

Yes____ No____

4- Accompanies you as a family to receive rehabilitative treatment:

Always _____ Sometimes _____ Never_____

5- You as a family apply some rehabilitative treatment at home:

Always _____ Sometimes _____ Never_____

6- Do you think he would improve if you, as a family, helped him in his rehabilitation treatment?

Yes _____ No _____.

Annex 3

Table 1

Distribution by sex of stroke patients in the rehabilitation room of the Omar Ranedo Pubillones Polyclinic.

Sex	Number of patients	%
Male	31	65.9
Female	16	34.0
Total	47	100

Annex 4

Table 2

Age and sex distribution of stroke patients.

Age(years)	Female		Male		Total	
	NO.	%	NO.	%	NO.	%
60	1	2.1	1	2.1	2	4.2
61	1	2.1	-	-	1	2.1
62	-	-	2	4.2	2	4.2
63	1	2.1	2	4.2	3	6.4
64	3	6.4	5	10.6	8	17
65	1	2.1	2	4.2	3	6.4
66	-	-	5	10.6	5	10.6
67	1	2.1	3	6.4	4	8.5
68	-	-	2	4.2	2	4.2
69	1	2.1	1	2.1	2	4.2
70	1	2.1	1	2.1	2	4.2
71	1	2.1	3	6.4	4	8.5
72	2	4.2	2	4.2	4	8.5
73	3	6.4	1	2.1	4	8.5
74	-	-	1	2.1	1	2.1
TOTA	**16**	**34**	**31**	**65.9**	**47**	**100**

Source: Admissions and discharges record book and Clinical Histories.

Annex 5

Table 5

Distribution of patients according to risk factors.

Risk factors	Male		Female	
	NO.	%	NO.	%
Arterial hypertension.	24	51	13	28
Heart disease.	20	42.5	11	23.4
Diabetes mellitus.	10	21.2	12	25.5
Sedentary lifestyle.	22	47	9	19.1
Alcohol ingestion (occasional)	31	66	-	-
Smoking.	16	34	7	15
Obesity.	-	-	4	8.5

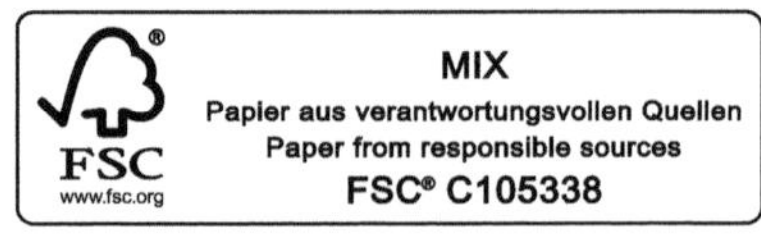

Printed by Books on Demand GmbH, Norderstedt / Germany